Nutrition for Beginners

What to Eat and Do to Live a Long and Happy Life

By: Crystal Stevens

Introduction

"Nutrition for Beginners: What to Eat and Do to Live a Long and Happy Life".

This book contains proven steps and strategies on how to eat right, live right, and stay happy and healthy throughout your life. Nutrition plays a big part of our lives, and we can't just live day by day, not knowing how good or bad the things we are consuming on a regular basis.

In today's modern times, everything around us is done instantly — instant coffee, instant noodles, instant rice, instant oatmeal, ready-to-eat meals, frozen foods, fast foods, as well as express delivery. People have become so preoccupied with a lot of things, that everything — including food and eating — has become fast paced.

We have mastered the art of multitasking, just so we can accommodate two or more things at a given time. Eating in front of the computer or consuming coffee while driving is not a skill anymore, but a habit. Gone are the days where people actually enjoy their meals with friends or tea time at the table, taking time to enjoy every bite and savor the exquisiteness of the food that they are eating.

For many people, things like career, education, adventure, and ambitions have become their priorities, even if it meant sacrificing the real "essentials" of life such as health, happiness, love, and social being. They ignore the real meaning of living a happy and healthy life because they are too focused on temporary pleasures and instant gratification brought by work, demanding activities, and material things.

With this modern lifestyle and trending habits, you may think that you're gaining time, wealth, or success. But the truth is, you are losing — losing nutrition, losing your health, losing opportunities to enjoy life. Think again. Is this really how you want to live your life?

If you want to live a long and happy life, you have to take action now! Ditch the wrong foods, change your lifestyle, and regain your health before it's too late.

I hope you enjoy it!

Chapter 1: The Importance of Good Nutrition

Nutrition plays a vital role in enabling us to live a happy and healthy life — free from worries, stress, diseases, and physical inconveniences.

As the popular adage says, "You are what you eat." This is true, because what you constantly put inside your body will show on the outside. You eat fattening foods, you get fat. You drink 5 cups of coffee in a day, you're awake and energized throughout the day. And when you eat healthy, nutritious foods religiously, you will achieve a lean, strong body that can counter illnesses and diseases.

Therefore, it is really important that you be mindful of what you constantly feed your body. Just because it's good to the taste doesn't mean it's good for your health. Similarly, not everything that is healthy and nutritious are delicious. You have to be aware of the nutritional content and value of each food you consume, because it will eventually define the quality of health you will possess.

This book will help you become more aware of the foods you regularly consume — what is good, what is bad, what you need to eat more, and what you need to avoid. If you are ready to take you health and your life to the next level, then continue reading. You will definitely see a different perspective on the foods you're eating afterwards.

What is Nutrition?

According to the World Health Organization, nutrition refers to the "intake of food, considered in relation to the body's dietary needs." Simply put, nutrition is what we eat and how the body uses the nutrients in the foods that we eat.

Nutrition also focuses on the role of healthy, well-balanced diet in preventing and managing diseases, conditions, and health problems. Similarly, it also involves identifying how certain conditions and illnesses may be caused by various dietary factors, including poor diet or malnutrition, food intolerances, sensitivities, and allergies.

WHO emphasizes that good nutrition is a cornerstone of good health, where they define good nutrition as an adequate, well-balanced diet combined with regular physical activity. Poor nutrition, on the other hand, can lead to increased susceptibility to diseases, weakened immunity, impaired physical and cognitive development, and reduced productivity.

Why Good Nutrition is Important?

What you choose to eat each day can affect your health today, tomorrow, and in the future. Good nutrition, therefore, is an important part of achieving a long life and a healthy lifestyle. Combined with regular exercises, your diet can contribute to maintaining a healthy weight, reducing risks of chronic diseases, and promoting overall wellness.

Below is a list of the importance of good nutrition that should motivate you to choose healthy foods every single time:

1. Eating the right food gives you energy. You body gets energy from the foods and drinks you consume. If the food you eat lacks the proper nutrient to fuel you, you may easily feel tired, irritable, or dehydrated.

2. Proper nutrition helps improve your immune system and protects your body from acquiring diseases. Foods that are high in vitamins and minerals and low in fats will support a healthy immune system.

3. The right choices of food can also help delay the effects of aging. Foods like tomatoes, avocados, fish, and nuts contain nutrients that are good for the skin and help build collagen.

Berries are high in vitamins and anti-oxidants that promote cell regeneration for new skin.

4. Healthy, home-cooked meals promote a long and happy life. Foods that are rich in nutrients and don't contain preservatives have been found to have a positive effect on life expectancy. On the other hand, fast foods and processed foods are full of harmful ingredients that are detrimental to your health.

5. Good nutrition improves your overall well-being. Healthy and nutritious foods are not only good for your physical body, but also promotes strong mental and emotional health.

These are the reasons why doctors, nutritionists, and health experts encourage proper nutrition to people of all ages. From babies to elderly, choosing the right kinds of foods — and eliminating the bad ones — are necessary in maintaining a healthy, well-balanced life.

Risks of Poor Nutrition

It may be easy to accept and agree to the many benefits of good nutrition to one's body, mind, and overall health. But are you aware of the risks and dangers of having a poor nutrition?

Many people turn to bad food choices due to lack of knowledge of what these bad foods can do to their health. For them, as long as something is edible or is accepted by their body, they can consume it for as long as they want. Moreover, a lot of individuals depend their food choices on taste, that if something is delicious or flavorful, it's automatically part of their daily meal plan, without even evaluating the nutritional value of that food.

These show wrong judgement of nutrition. If you continue to consume food based on taste, unhealthy preferences, or just because it's "popular" in the market, you are going towards the route of poor nutrition.

Having poor nutrition or unhealthy food choices is harmful to your health. You may not experience the danger now, but the negative effects will surely show up in the future, when it's already late to take actions. Some of the risks and dangers of poor nutrition include the following:

- Being obese or overweight
- High blood pressure
- High cholesterol
- Heart diseases and stroke
- Eating disorders and digestive problems
- Tooth decay
- Type 2 diabetes
- Hepatitis
- Osteoporosis
- Some types of cancers

It is, therefore, important to start taking action now than later. If you are aware that your food choices are not the most ideal ones, then it's time to make some changes and improve your diet. In the next chapter, you will learn which specific food items, products, and ingredients should you include in your diet, and which ones should you ditch.

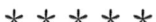

CHAPTER SUMMARY:

- Nutrition plays a vital role in the kind of life you will have now, tomorrow, and in the future.

- According to the World Health Organization, nutrition refers to the intake of food, considered in relation to the body's dietary needs.

- The importance of good nutrition includes giving the body energy it needs, improving your immune system, delaying the effects of aging, promoting a long and happy life, and improve your overall well-being.

- On the other hand, poor nutrition can lead to a number of health concerns and problems, including obesity, high blood pressure, high cholesterol, heart diseases, stroke, cancers, diabetes, osteoporosis, and more.

Chapter 2: 10 Essential Nutrition Tips for Beginners

From the previous chapter, we have established that good nutrition plays a vital role in achieving a healthy body and preventing health-related diseases. In this chapter, we will discuss what specific food items, products, and ingredients that you should consume and how they can boost your physical, mental, and emotional health.

Similarly, we will also talk about the specific foods and drinks that are detrimental to your health. These will be discussed, not to encourage or tolerate you to consume them, but to make you realize the harmful effects they bring to your body and health.

1. Reduce Sugar Intake

People need glucose – in the form of sugar – daily for energy. But before putting that chocolate or pastry in your mouth, know first that consuming too much sugar or sweet foods will not only destroy your teeth, but will lead to so much weight gain, as well. So, make sure to take in only the right amount of sugar needed by your body. For male, the recommended sugar intake is 150 calories or 9 teaspoons, and for female, it's 100 calories or 6 teaspoons.

Also, remember that sugar does not refer only to cakes, chocolates, and candies. The body can get the needed dose of sugar through healthy food like bread, potatoes, rice, and vegetables.

To reduce sugar intake and keep your body healthy, follow these simple diet tips:

- Instead of heaping that sugar on your coffee or juice, switch to low-calorie sweeteners available in granulated form, sachets, and tablets.

- Limit the sugar you use in cooking. If available, consider using low-calorie sweeteners for cooking, baking, and sprinkling.

- Reduce your intake of processed or canned foods since most of these products contain hidden sugar.

- As much as possible, eat sugar-free or low sugar food.

- Instead of indulging in cakes, ice creams, and other high-caloric sweets, you can get a dose of your needed sugar by eating healthier foods like fruits, potatoes, pastas, and cereals.

- Between meals, avoid frizzy or fruit drinks as they can cause tooth decay. Instead, snack on fruits, low-fat yogurt, or low-sugar cereal products.

Remember the adage too much of anything is bad? This does not exempt sugar intake. So, before you get diagnosed with high blood sugar or diabetes, start controlling your sugar intake and opt for a healthier and sweeter life.

2. Eat Fiber-Rich Foods

Fiber plays an essential role in maintaining good health. People who eat fiber-rich foods are taking good care of their heart. Fiber is useful in keeping the heart healthy as it washes out bad cholesterol from saturated fat that keeps clogging blood vessels and arteries. Moreover, fiber provides an easy, safes and affordable means of reducing blood pressure in patients with hypertension.

Nutritionists suggest that daily fiber intake must be 25 to 30 grams per day on a 2,000-calorie diet for adults. A cupful of quick cook oatmeal or whole wheat toast is already enough for a day's fiber treat. On other days, you can try fixing fiber-rich serving of tossed salad with low-fat dressing or bran muffins with soft, low-fat margarine.

Fruits and vegetables are the best sources of fiber in foods. Fresh cranberries are not only rich in fiber, but taste good and contain good antioxidants for the body, as well. If fresh cranberries aren't available at your local market, you can substitute fresh cranberry fruit juice and yogurt for a delicious and healthy fiber intake.

Other fiber-rich sources include wheat, dried beans and peas, whole-wheat pasta, brown rice, and whole-grain breads and cereals. So, before munching on any snack, read the labels first and make sure that it contains high content of fiber.

3. Munch on High-Protein Meals

Protein is essential in repairing impaired tissues from our day-to-day physical activities and building new muscles in the body. This is why nutritionists and experts recommend high-protein foods for athletes, sports enthusiasts, and gym buffs.

However, whether you're working out on a regular basis or not, you still need to consume a good amount of protein everyday. Eating protein with low fat content will not only help you control your weight, but also keeps your heart healthy.

Food rich in protein include poultry (skinless), low-fat or fat-free dairy products (yogurt, milk and cheese), fish, and plant proteins which include beans, tofu, soy milk and dried peas. Make sure to include a significant amount of protein-rich food in your meals.

4. Double Up Your Daily Dose of Veggies

Make the vegetable portions on your dinner plate twice the size of your meat portion. Mother Nature's gems, vegetables, are full of vitamins, minerals, and fiber, and typically, low in fat and heart-unhealthy, saturated fat. More importantly, high bulks, low-calorie veggies fill you up before they fill you out, crowding out the opportunity to overeat the higher fat meats at dinner.

To stave off the mid-afternoon hungry horrors, tack on some veggies at lunch to create a more satisfying, higher volume mid-day meal. Add a side salad with your sandwich or stuff a salad into a whole wheat pita along with some lean protein. If cold veggies at lunch make you shiver, brew a pot of vegetable soup and slurp it up along with your lunch sandwich.

Eating three to five servings of veggies daily can help appease your hunger, yet please your waist. Keep your meat to no more than 3-ounces (about the size of a woman's palm) at dinner and double up on the veggies on your plate.

5. Make Gains with Whole Grains

Digestible carbohydrates including sugar, white flour, and other highly processed starches increase cancer risk. In one study, women who ate the most non-fiber carbohydrates increased their risk of colon cancer almost seven times over that of women who ate the least amount. Men who ate the most also doubled their risk of cancer of the rectum.

But here comes the good news. A switch to whole grains may have the opposite effect. The term "whole" is a tip-off to getting a whole lot more nutrition. Research shows rye bread can improve your bowel movements and may lower the concentration of some cancer-causing compounds in your colon.

What's more, oat and whole wheat breads – whether plain or toasted – are good for the colon. You can also benefit if you eat corn and barley for their resistant starch. And to top it all off, studies have shown that wheat bran can inhibit both colon and intestinal tumors better than other bran types such as oat or barley. A wheat bran cereal is a convenient way to add this cancer fighter to your day.

So, take every opportunity to replace those processed carbohydrates with whole grains. You may like the hearty taste of whole grains a whole lot better, and your bowels may benefit, too.

6. Be Finicky about Fats and Oils

Avoid unhealthy fats at all cost. Fat raises cancer risk. In fact, European researchers found that red meat, processed meat in particular, increases the risk of colon cancer.

Look out for saturated and trans fat because they are unhealthy for the heart. Fatty foods are not only high in calories, but will also make you gain a lot of weight. Limit your intake of oil, cream, cheese, bacon, ice cream, red meats, baked sweet goods, butter, and margarine as they contain unhealthy fats that are not good for the heart.

Start replacing red meat and cheeses with lower-fat alternatives such as fish, poultry, and beans. Use low-fat cooking methods like baking and broiling, too. Look for other ways to lower fat such as choosing no-fat and low-fat snacks. What's more, if you give up snack foods that are fried at high temperatures such as potato chips and french fries, you will also give up a source of acrylamide, a possible cancer-causing compound.

Moreover, do not forget to choose your oils carefully. Fish oil and olive oil can help you against colon cancer, while corn oil may actually raise your risk.

7. Drink Less Juice and Eat More Fruits

To get the full benefits of foods especially fruits, eat them whole instead of juicing them. Eating the fruit whole lets you intake the maximum nutrients the fruit can offer without wasting some necessary elements.

Fruits, when peeled or cut and extracted of its juice for drinking, lose some of the important dietary fibers that they are most useful for. They get discarded with the peeling.

Extracting the juice of the fruits to ingest its nutrients by drinking may also let you exceed your sugar and other nutrients requirements. Let's take orange as an example. It takes at least four medium oranges to make a glassful of orange juice, depending on how juicy the oranges are. A medium size orange can have as much as 12 grams of sugar or the equivalent caloric value of 48 calories. Do the math and you will realize how four or more oranges can shoot your sugar and calorie intake up which is not good for your weight loss program. Also, the increase in other nutrients like vitamins and minerals, is not always good. An orange already contains twice your daily Vitamin C need.

8. Avoid Fast Foods and Processed Foods

Commercially processed foods not only lack the proper nutrients your body needs; they are also detrimental to your health if you keep consuming them regularly. Canned baked beans, instant soups and noodles, ketchup, canned luncheon meats, processed corned beefs, and barbecue sauces are just a few examples of processed foods that you may be stocking in your pantry cabinet.

Fast foods are just as unhealthy as processed foods. Foods sold at fast foods contain lots of calories, because they are mainly made up of carbohydrates and unhealthy fat and only a few amount of protein. This is exactly the reverse of the proportion which a person should actually consume. This ration of carbohydrates and protein, if kept at a steady pace, will eventually cause the arteries to get clogged, leading to many cardiovascular problems.

Both processed and fast foods can be described as tasty, because they were designed that way to entice your taste buds and make you want them more. No wonder you keep eating them again and again.

But being tasty is not the same as being nutritious. The flavor of processed foods and fast foods are enhanced with the addition of sugar, salt, and other condiments beyond their healthy limits. What's more, many condiments put on these types of foods like ketchup and sauces such as spaghetti sauce and barbecue sauce are, by themselves, unhealthy, owing to high sugar and salt contents.

9. Regulate Salt Intake

Salt is a chemical compound that our body needs as it helps to regulate blood volume and pressure. Our body requires both sodium and chloride, but it cannot manufacture these elements on its own. Therefore, we get these nutrients from our food. However, it is important to regulate our intake of salt. Many studies have shown that decreasing or increasing salt intake can have a direct impact on blood pressure.

Keeping to 2,400 mg of sodium a day is doable. This is because about 75% of the sodium in our diet comes from processed foods and just 10% comes from the saltshaker. Make it a habit to check food labels and try to eat food with less than 200 mg of sodium per serving. Avoid high-sodium foods that have more than 800 mg per serving.

Do not attempt to eliminate salt in your diet – it is essential and required by the body. Instead, try to reduce excessive intake by consuming whole, unprocessed foods and minimizing the amount of salt that you add to meals.

10. Dose Up in Vitamin C

Vitamin C, also known as ascorbic acid, is one of the body's most effective defenses against ailments. It fortifies the immune system for stronger resistance against different infections. It also keeps dental tissues tight and fit, thus, keeping gums and teeth strong and healthy.

Vitamin C is also essential in keeping the cement-like matter between cells strong and prevents cataracts and other eye diseases. It hastens the repair of cuts and wounds and keeps the bones strong.

The rich sources of this water-soluble vitamin are fresh fruits and vegetables. Citrus fruits are the best sources of Vitamin C like lime, orange, pomelo, and naranjita. Non-citrus fruits like guavas, papayas, tomatoes, and chicos are also high in Vitamin C. Also, vegetables like mongo sprouts and bamboo shoots contain Vitamin C.

BONUS TIP! Drink at least two liters of water daily.

Water is one of the most important things that are needed to sustain life on earth. It is categorized as nutrient for without water, every single function of our body will become dehydrated and thus may cause serious illness or death.

It serves as the carrier of nutrients and oxygen to all parts of the body and regulates body temperature. And since our body loses water through perspiration, urination, and respiration, it is advisable to drink at least two liters of water or eight eight-ounce glasses of water daily. The more, the better.

If you drink alcohol or coffee, drink an equal amount of water. When exercising, drink another glass for every 20 minutes of physical exertion. Not only does water replenish the lost liquid in your body, it also makes you feel full faster, thus preventing you from snacking on unhealthy treats.

* * * * *

CHAPTER SUMMARY:

- If you are just starting to improve your diet and food choices, there are basic nutrition tips you need to keep in mind in order to achieve proper nutrition. These include the following:

  - Reduce sugar intake. Consume only the right amount of sugar needed by your body daily.

  - Eat fiber-rich foods, including fruits, vegetables, wheat, dried beans, whole-wheat pasta, brown rice, whole-grain breads and cereals.

  - Make protein-rich foods part of your meals, such as eggs, chicken, fish, and plant-based foods.

  - Make the vegetable portions on your dinner plate twice the size of your meat portion.

  - Make a switch from consuming processed carbohydrates to eating whole grains.

  - Choose healthy fats and oils, especially when used in cooking and preparing foods.

  - Make it a habit to eat the whole fruit instead of drinking only its juice to get the full benefits.

  - Avoid fast foods and processed foods at all costs. It is better to prepare home-cooked meals to ensure that you're getting the full nutrition from your foods.

  - Regulate salt intake. Reduce excessive intake by consuming whole, unprocessed foods and minimizing the amount of salt that you add to meals.

- Dose up in vitamin C as it is one of the body's most effective defenses against ailments.

- Finally, make sure that you drink at least 2 liters of water everyday to keep you hydrated and replenish lost liquids in your body.

Chapter 3: A Quick Look at Food Supplements

You may have heard about various food supplements and their corresponding benefits to the human body. But are they essential to good health? Do we need to take in food supplements in order to reach that "quality of life" that we've always wanted? This chapter shall discuss about food supplements and their vital role in human health.

What are Food Supplements?

Also known as dietary supplements, food supplements contain essential substances including vitamins, minerals, or amino acids that are helpful to the human body. As the name suggests, food supplements contain specific dietary ingredients that "supplement" or add to the nutrients that you are giving your body through the food you eat. However, these supplements are not formulated to substitute a real meal.

People generally take food supplements to fulfill a specific health requirement. For example, if you advised to consume 1000mg of Calcium a day, but you are only able to eat foods that contain 400mg of Calcium, you may want to add more to this dietary requirement by taking in a Calcium supplement. It is important to know that food supplements are merely for boosting specific nutrients in the body, and should not be used as an alternative to traditional curative medicines.

While food supplements do not cure or treat specific illnesses, they can, however, contribute to improving health and over well-being of the individual. Similar to other forms of alternative medicines, food supplements are preventive in nature.

The Need for Food Supplements

After getting a pretty clear idea what food supplements are and what they do for the body, the next questions would probably be who needs to take them? Are food supplements meant for everyone? Or are they only for those possessing bad health conditions?

Food supplements are for everyone. No exceptions.

According to Annette Dickinson, Ph.D. and a member of the Council for Responsible Nutrition on her study entitled Who Needs Supplements: Most people Have Nutrition Gaps that Supplements Can Fill published in June 2002, nutritional supplementation is recommended for adults. Appropriate supplementation can be determined on the basis of a person's age, gender, and dietary patterns, without the need for individual screening.

Even the healthiest-looking individuals are advised to take food and dietary supplements for many reasons. Below are some of the reasons why we should not depend entirely on the food we eat and, therefore, take food supplements in achieving optimal health.

1. **Soil depletion reduces the nutrient content of our food supply.** In many areas of the world, the land in which food are planted and harvested has been over-farmed and overgrazed. This means that manures and other mineral-rich products are not put back enough on the land, depleting the quality of the soil. This produces food that is low in minerals, vitamins, and hundreds of other nutrients.

2. **The use of modern fertilizers does not provide enough trace elements.** Trace elements, also known as micronutrients, form part of a person's daily diet, and play a vital role in maintaining his health, vitality, and well-being.

One hundred years ago, manures were used extensively for fertilizer and effectively preserve the nutrition of food. Nowadays, superphosphate fertilizers are being used to replace manures. Containing nitrogen, potassium, and phosphorus primarily, they do not supply enough in trace elements. Hence, harvested crops are artificially stimulated or enhanced, but not as nutritious and safe.

3. **Hybrid crops provide fewer nutrients.** To provide sufficient supply of crops to the ever increasing population of the world, farmers have no choice but to enforce hybrid planting. With this approach, at least ten times as much rice or wheat, for example, are grown on the same land as was grown there a hundred years ago. This land, however, is not stocked with ten times the vitamins, minerals, and other nutrients. As a result, today's wheat contains only about 6% protein compared to 12-14% 100 years ago. Trace mineral levels are similarly much lower due to high-yield farming methods.

4. **The use of chemical pesticides and herbicides increase toxicity level in food.** Many pesticides being used in farming and harvesting are deadly chemicals that severely destroy the human system. Some even contain lead, arsenic, and other toxic metals that slowly accumulate in the body.

5. **The transportation of food reduces their nutritional content.** The levels of certain nutrients in food begin to diminish as soon as it is harvested. Today, many foods are grown thousands of miles from their designated markets and population centers. Some of the foods we buy from the market or grocery store actually spent a week on a truck or a train.

6. **Processing of food lessens their nutritional content.** Among the foods or ingredients affected by this include rice, dairy products, and wheat flour. For example, when wheat is refined to make white flour, 80% of magnesium, 70-80% of zinc, 87% of chromium, 88% of manganese and 50% of cobalt get removed instantaneously. Similarly, refining sugar cane to produce white sugar removes 99% of magnesium and 93% of its chromium.

7. **Poor eating habits weaken the absorption of nutrients.** Skipping meals, binge eating, and high level of alcohol consumption are just some of the negative eating habits that most people today are doing. Due to bad habits and poor quality of food, most people do not absorb nutrients well at all. This impairs nutrient levels in the body, and increases nutritional needs.

8. **Stressful lifestyle impairs digestion.** When the body is stressed, exhausted, and always in a hurry, certain nutrients are being used up more, including calcium, zinc, magnesium, chromium, manganese and many others, and this gets eliminated from the body. Stress adds to all the other causes of impaired nutrition and becomes a source of excessive sympathetic nervous system activity. This, in turn, reduces nutrient absorption and utilization even further.

Food supplements will, therefore, restore or bring back the nutrients that have been reduced, removed, and totally eliminated from the conditions identified above. It is then important to identify what nutrients your body needs to attain optimal health.

Similar to other traditional medicines, before consuming any type of food supplements, be sure to check first with your doctor.

* * * * *

CHAPTER SUMMARY:

- Food supplements are substances that contain essential ingredients needed by the body to function well. They work by "supplementing" or adding to the nutrients that you are giving your body through the food you eat.

- Food supplements are usually taken to fulfill a specific health requirement, especially if one cannot consume the entire amount of a natural substance on a regular basis.

- There are several reasons why you need to supplement your food, especially if the nutrients in them have been depleted lost.

Chapter 4: Other Tips for a Long and Happy Life

Nutrition is just one part of the formula for a long, happy, and healthy life. By knowing what you need to eat and consuming only the healthy variants of food, you are nourishing your mind and body with the right nutrients that they need in order to function well.

More than a having a healthy body and mind, if your goal is to live live a long and happy life, there are other things you need to do and practices you need to follow. Here are other important factors that contribute to acquiring maximum health and wellness.

Eliminate Stress from Your Life

Stress not only causes emotional threat, it can also negatively affect your physical and mental health. Therefore, if you want to have a nice, peaceful life, you need to get rid of stress right now!

Experiencing a little stress once in a while is normal, but if you get to the point where you can't handle it and it becomes long term, stress can seriously affect your life, job, family, and health negatively. According to a survey, more than half of Americans admit that they fight with their loved ones and friends when they get stressed. Further more, more than 70% share that they experience emotional and physical symptoms because of stress.

When left unmanaged, stress can contribute to a number of health problems, including high blood pressure, diabetes, obesity, and heart diseases. It can also lead to emotional troubles like irritability, sleep problems, and depression.

To reduce, if not totally eliminate, stress from your life, here are some effective ways you can do:

- Practice meditation and mindfulness. Everyday, spend 5 to 10 minutes alone to meditate and pay attention to your life and surroundings. You can repeatedly say a mantra in your mind while taking slow deep breaths.

- Relax and try guided imagery. Whenever you start feeling bothered by external factors like traffic, noise, or toxic people, step back for awhile and close your eyes. Relax your body and mind, while picturing yourself in a "happy place". Guided imagery can be very effective in pulling you away from stressful situations and bringing you to a peaceful place.

- Focus on breathing. Proper breathing techniques can quickly calm your body and brain. To do these, breathe in through your nose, while slowly counting to three. Hold your breath for one second, and then slowly breathe out through your nose while counting again to three.

- Engage in aromatherapy. Aromatherapy has been proven to provide stress relief, and helps you feel more relaxed, energized, and focused in the moment. Some researches even report that certain scents can modify brain wave activities and significantly reduce stress hormones in the body.

- Travel and make time for leisure activities. When work, house chores, business deals, or school gets stressful, take time to engage in leisure activities like shopping, spending time with friends, going for a long walk, playing sports, or traveling to a new place. Injecting some leisure time in your day or week can help you feel and perform better.

Eliminate stress now and be on your way to a happy, peaceful, and comfortable life.

Engage in Exercises and Physical Activities

Staying active is essential in achieving a happy, healthy, and long life. This is because exercises and physical activities help strengthen your heart enable proper blood circulation, making you feel better, more energized, and more relaxed.

Additionally, when you engage in regular exercises and physical activities, you can lower your risk of certain health conditions, including heart attack, obesity, high blood pressure, osteoporosis, and more. It can also help you manage your weight better, develop stronger bones and muscles, and recover faster from hospitalizations or bed rest.

Regularly engaging in physical exercises doesn't mean you need to spend hours in the gym day after day after day. You can play your favorite sports or indulge in something you enjoy like bowling, swimming, or jogging around the park. Also, when you spending most of your day sitting on the couch or in front of the computer, make sure that you take frequent breaks to do quick stretching, take a quick walk, or climb up and down the stairs, just to loosen up your joints and muscles.

Quit Cigarettes, Alcoholic Drinks, and Drugs Now

Despite the known fact and figures that cigarettes, alcohol, and drugs can dramatically harm your physical and mental health, many people still turn to these substances just because, according to them, these vices make them feel good about themselves — temporarily. According to a report from the National Survey on Drug Use and Health (NSDUH), in the United States alone, almost 20 million Americans over the age of 12 suffered from substance use disorder in 2017. Almost 74% of these individuals also struggled with alcohol abuse.

From the National Institute on Alcohol Abuse and Alcoholism, tobacco is the leading preventable cause of death in the United States, while alcohol ranks third. It is alarming that people as young as 12 years old are already exposed to these substances that may actually lead them to their deaths.

Aside from deaths, injuries, and disabilities, these harmful substances cause a wide array of physical and mental health problems, as well, including cancer of different types, tuberculosis, heart diseases, high blood pressure, digestive problems, pancreatitis, liver cirrhosis, liver cancer, and various psychological conditions. Additionally, they can also cause seizures, stroke, memory problems, mental confusion, and brain damage.

If you let yourself get trapped, abused, and addicted to one or all of these substances, it may be difficult to live normally and healthily. Therefore, if you want to live a long and happy life, free from negative effects of these substances, then quit now... before it's too late.

Get at Least 8 Hours of Sleep Every Night

Getting good quality and complete sleep every night is essential as it helps relax, recharge, and rejuvenate the body and mind, especially after a tiring or stressful day. During this time, your body also heals damaged cells and tissues. As you sleep, there is increased blood supply to the muscles which helps in the repair of such muscles. The increased secretions of growth hormones by the pituitary glands promote tissue growth and repair. Also, sleep builds our immunity to infection.

On the other hand, lack of sleep, affects memory storage and retention adversely. It reduces immunity to infection and diseases. It makes the body's reaction time slower and concentration, and analysis harder. It induces a feeling of lethargy and mood shifts, producing high level of stress and anxiety during the day. If your body continuously gets less sleep than you need, the effect is cumulative. There is a need to make up for the lost hours of sleep for the body to recover from the loss.

To help you get achieve quality and enough sleep every night, try the following approaches.

- Schedule your sleep. Go to bed at the same time every night and train your biological time to wake at the same time every morning even during the weekends or holidays. This would establish your sleep cycle. It also means that you get the same number of sleep every night.

- Reduce caffeine and alcohol before bedtime. The chemicals introduced to the body by bad habit such as smoking, drinking and too much caffeine disrupt the body's natural rhythm, making it harder to establish a regular sleep schedule.

- If you're having trouble sleeping, try meditation, aromatherapy, warm shower, and a soft massage before going to bed. Additionally, avoid too much screen time before sleeping as it stimulates your brain further and prevents you from falling asleep right away.

Cultivate a Positive Attitude

In today's world full of cruelty, depressing news, and violence, a positive attitude is a breathe of fresh air. Many benefits can be traced from having a positive mind and attitude, including success and happiness. This is caused by the fact that positive thinking can push you to work hard and strive for your goals, preventing minor problems from getting in the way.

If you cultivate a positive mindset, you are not letting negative thoughts, actions, and events bring you down. You are focusing your mind to the more important things, rather than worrying about the things you cannot control. You tend to be more mindful to other people's feelings and actions. You become kinder, gentler, and happier.

According to Gertrude Weaver, who died at the age of 116 in Arkansas, her longevity is due to her "kindness". When she was interviewed by Time Magazine upon claiming the title "world's oldest woman", she advised, "treat people right and be nice to other people the way you want them to be nice to you." No matter how cliche this sounds, a research done at the University of North Carolina affirms that positive thinking contributes to a person's health, while negativity and stress can be detrimental.

* * * * *

CHAPTER SUMMARY:

- While good nutrition and consuming the right types of food are essential in achieving a healthy life, there are other important factors that contribute to living a long and happy life.

- Reducing or eliminating stress from your life is one of these factors. Stress can negatively affect your life, career, family, and health, so it's important to take control of the things that stress you out.

- Engaging in regular exercises, physical activities, and sports can also contribute to a long and happy life. Move more and perform activities that your enjoy.

- Cigarette smoking, alcohol, and drug abuse are detrimental to one's health and life. Therefore, you need to avoid these substances if you want to live happily and healthily.

- Moreover, getting enough sleep every night and cultivating a positive attitude are also necessary in achieving a life that is free from worries, diseases, and things that can weigh you down.

Conclusion

I hope this book was able to help you to realize the importance of good nutrition and how it contributes to achieving a long, happy, and healthy life. If you used to just eat to your heart's — and stomach's — content without thinking about the consequences to your health, now is the time to make a change and level up your health.

The next step is to take action and improve your eating habits. I understand that it may not be easy at the start and you may need to make a lot of adjustments. But if keep your eye to your goal, which is to create a healthier and longer life, you will do what it takes to keep going.

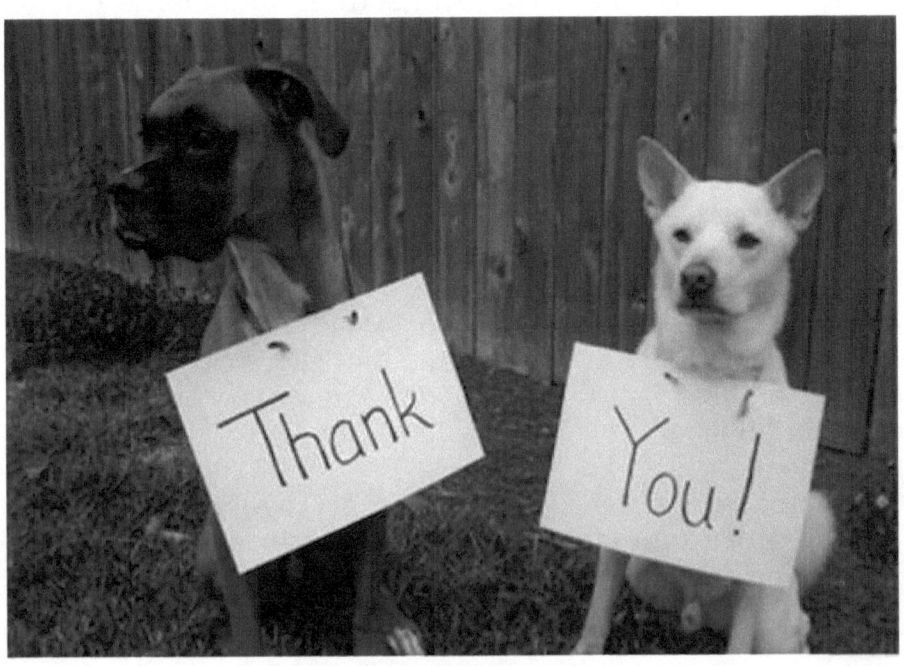

So, if you enjoyed this book, I'd like to ask you for a favor. Would you be kind enough to leave a review for this book on Amazon? It'd be greatly appreciated!

Thank you and good luck!

www.ingramcontent.com/pod-product-compliance
Lightning Source LLC
Chambersburg PA
CBHW051406280526
45784CB00007B/3121